Cypress Essential Oil

Benefits, Properties, Applications, Studies & Recipes

by Ann Sullivan

Published in USA by:

Ann Sullivan
217 N. Seacrest Blvd #9
Boynton Beach
FL 33425

© Copyright 2016

ISBN-13: ISBN-13: 978-1544755557
ISBN-10: ISBN-10: 1544755554

Table of Contents

Introduction

What are essential oils and how might they be used for therapeutic purposes?

Essential oils are ultra-potent oils extracted from plants and flowers that have been utilized in medicine for centuries. Presently, they are most commonly used to supplement pharmaceutical medication, but they can also be an effective alternative to pharmaceuticals in the event that there is no access to them. Before dismissing essential oils as a means to support the body's natural defenses against injury and illness, take a look at the historical evidence of the oils' therapeutic competence in practice. The average age-old medical text will demonstrate that essential oils, herbs, and plenty of other natural ingredients have, for thousands of years, successfully enhanced immune function to meet and defeat any number of ailments and injuries. Though traditional medicine is considered "alternative" now, it was once the gold standard. Perhaps it still should be, as these natural age-tested remedies can fortify the body's defenses against everything from simple maladies, like headaches, cuts, and bruises to serious diseases, like cancer.

Essential oils are deemed "essential," because the oils are composed of the "essence" of the plant. The difference between essential oils and other oils – like olive oil or vegetable oil, for instance – is that essential oils have high volatility and reduced fixation, which results in faster evaporation, enabling their popular use in aromatherapy. Even at high temperatures, olive and vegetable oils do not evaporate.

Essential oils are especially necessary when it comes to a major natural or man-made disaster or potential viral outbreak. In these dire situations, people may not have quick access to their standard pharmaceutical supply; so, essential oils, along with other alternative medicines, will be the go-to wellness aids in the case of social collapse, viral outbreak, or devastating natural disaster. When medical access is unavailable, alternatives to our modern-day standard are the only chance we have to keep pathogens at bay.

Most people do not realize that they already use essential oils every day. They are in perfumes, shampoos, soaps, and ointments; they are even used in furniture polish. Why are they found in so many aromatic products? Well, because essential oils are super concentrated aromatic liquids, so their scent is remarkably strong. Let us put this into perspective: to steam tea, use a few leaves of peppermint or juniper; to produce a single ounce of essential oil, five whole *pounds* of peppermint or juniper leaves are required. Some sources claim that to produce twelve pounds of essential oil would necessitate an acre of peppermint, juniper, or any other oil being produced en masse. Unlike vegetable oil, you do not often find concentrated therapeutic-grade essential oils sold in bulk; instead the oils are often sold in easily carried small, dark bottles, perfect for the GOOD bag (Get Out Of Dodge). That is exactly what this book is aiming to help people plan for – getting out of dodge with the most vital of essential oils intact, a good supply of Cypress essential oil.

Why Cypress, you ask? Well, to get quickly up to speed on this most essential of oils, below we have provided a condensed synopsis of Cypress, after which we will outline in greater detail the oil's history, properties, and common therapeutic uses, so that you – the consumer – might have a better understanding of the oil's benefits and applications. We have even provided supportive remedies for pure Cypress, as well as blended recipes that incorporate the valuable oil. Chapter 3 will further detail past scientific research on Cypress essential oil.

Now, let's get down to it. **Essential Oil 101: The Basics of Cypress**

Summary: Cypress, or Cypressus sempervirens, has been used for thousands of years to combat various conditions. Primarily, the oil's circulatory properties made it a go-to support for menstrual issues, as it helped to regulate blood flow. Those same properties help decrease water retention, ease muscle tension, and detox the lymphatic system. Cypress is also said to alleviate fear of change and promote a feeling of inner security.

Description: Cypress oil is commonly extracted through steam distillation. The needles are most often used. The oil is often pale yellow in color, thin in consistency, and has a medium natural and woody scent.

Uses: Beyond those applications previously mentioned, additional uses for Cypress essential oil include strengthening the body's defenses against bronchitis, the lymphatic system, arthritis, poor circulation, diabetes, menopausal issues, prostate, rheumatism, throat issues, cramps, insomnia, pancreas insufficiencies, pulmonary tuberculosis, spasms, varicose veins, oily skin and hair, hemorrhoids, and menorrhagia. Cypress also reduces perspiration and water retention. The oil can mentally ground the user, making them feel increasingly secure and confident.

Properties: Antioxidant, antibacterial, antifungal, anti-inflammatory, cytotoxic, sudorific, anti-infectious, sedative, antiseptic, astringent, antispasmodic, decongestant, vasoconstrictor, diuretic, hemostatic, hepatic, and mucolytic properties.

Application: Dilute 1:1 with a carrier oil. You can apply topically or diffuse.

Safety Precautions: If pregnant or diabetic, consult a physician before using this oil. If you have sensitive skin, dilute heavily. Do not take internally.

Fun facts: Derived from the Greek word "sempervivens," meaning "live forever," Cypress promotes a long, healthy life. Ironically, Cypress shortened many a convicted criminal's life at the turn of the century, as crosses were often constructed of Cypress wood, including the cross that Jesus bore.

The religious connotations of this immortal wood don't end there – Greeks, as well, would carve their immortal gods out of wood, creating colorful statues. The wood's ties to the Roman God of the Underworld – the god who, in Greece, is known as Hades, the God of Death – reinforce the connection between Cypress and the transformative nature of the mind when faced with the unknown

Chapter 1:
Benefits of Cypress Essential Oil

Cypress essential oil offers several therapeutic benefits; but you may be wondering what these benefits are. In this chapter, we'll take a closer look at the history of Cypress and its many uses.

Cultivation of Cypress

Cypress, or Cypressus sempervirens, is a coniferous evergreen that can live for more than a thousand years and grows only to a median height of around 115 feet. The conic crown of the tree has branches that are level and hang, variable in length, and loosely. The foliage is dark green and grows densely with leaves that are 2-5 mm long and scaly with oblong seed cones that are 25-40 mm in length and mature to a brown color around two years following pollination.

The Cypress is cultivated across the Mediterranean and outside its native region as an ornamental tree. It thrives in climates that are mild and rainy in the winter and hot and dry in the summer, but it can also grow in areas with cool and humid summers. The Mediterranean Cypress has been brought to southern Australia, New Zealand, the British Isles, and South Africa, as well as California, Washington, Oregon, Florida, and British Columbia.

A History of Cypress

The Cypress tree, or Cypressus sempervirens, is also known as the graveyard Cypress, the Mediterranean Cypress, the Italian Cypress, or the Tuscan Cypress. This Cypress species grows in northeast Libya, northern Egypt, southern Albania, southern Turkey, southern Croatia, southeast Greece, western Syria, western Jordan, Cyprus, Israel, Italy, Lebanon, Malta, and the greater eastern Mediterranean region. Sempervirens, this Cypress species name, is derived from the Latin for 'evergreen'.

The essential oils from the Cypress tree are used in perfumery and cosmetics, due to the oil's scent, as well as its anti-aging, astringent, firming, and anti-dandruff properties. The Cypress is also renowned for its sturdy and aromatic wood. In fact, St. Peter's Basilica in Vatican City boasts doors made of Cypress. The wood is so strong that it stood the place of stainless steel before the metal was invented; it was used as staves to contain mash ferments for alcohol production in distilleries. Though sturdy, the tree is also flexible and offers a bit of drama on the horizon, due to its swaying in the lightest of breezes. In some regions, it's called the "drama tree."

Clocking in at around 4,000 years old, Sarv-e-Abarkooh, of Iran's Yazd Province, is the oldest living Cypress in the world. The ancient Cypresses of Iran were, and still are, the primary choice for gardens around the region, and are found in many of the famous Persian Gardens, marking a key design element in Dowlat-Abad and Fin Garden, for example.

The Cypress was such a significant element in classical antiquity that it symbolized mourning in both European culture and in the cultures of many Muslim countries. Because the Cypress often refuses to regrow when damaged or cut, the tree gained an association with death and the underworld, which has made it a mainstay in cemeteries, including the famous Turkish cemetery, Istanbul Karacaahmet Cemetery. Cypress was often made into garlands and hung around households in Athens when a member of the household had passed away. Statues of Pluto, the god of the underworld, were also adorned with Cypress garlands. Moreover, during cremations, the tree served to fumigate the air.

This association with death is also alluded to in a story by the poet, Ovid, who was alive during Augustus' rule. In this story, Apollo's favorite young boy, named Cyparissus, killed a stag by accident. This stag was the boy's pet and he had loved the animal so much that he grieved over it and was so remorseful that he wished to cry eternally. And so, the boy was turned into the Cypress tree and now his eternal tears continue to weep as the tree's sap.

Chemical Components

To generate the essential oil from Cypress, the needles must be steam distilled. This results in the oil's key chemical components, which are primarily linalool, alpha and beta pinene, terpinolene, bornyl acetate, myrcene, cadinene, alpha terpinene, cedrol, carene, sabinene, and camphene.

Main Properties of Cypress Essential Oil

Along with the properties previously mentioned in the introduction, Cypress oil possesses antioxidant, antibacterial, antifungal, anti-inflammatory, cytotoxic, sudorific, anti-infectious, sedative, antiseptic, astringent, antispasmodic, decongestant, vasoconstrictor, diuretic, hemostatic, hepatic, and mucolytic properties. With such a versatile range, Cypress is well equipped to fight off any pathogen in the body's path.

The oil, as mentioned, is composed of linalool, alpha and beta pinene, terpinolene, bornyl acetate, myrcene, cadinene, alpha terpinene, cedrol, carene, sabinene, and camphene. These components are what instill the enormously beneficial properties within Cypress essential oil. We'll outline these properties below.

Antioxidant

Anything high in antioxidants – whether fruit, beans, or essential oils – is a powerful advocate for your body. Antioxidants both protect against free radicals and repair their damage. What are free radicals? Free radicals are destructive chemicals that invade your body, produced by substances both inside and out. Some free radicals (or oxidants) form through normal bodily reactions, like inflammation, metabolism and aerobic respiration. Other free radicals form outside the body, but enter it due to exposure. These include harmful pollutants, toxins, smoking, alcohol, X-rays, and UV rays, to name a few. Although our bodies produce their own antioxidants, these often become damaged as we grow older; thus, introducing antioxidants into our bodies allows these nutrients and enzymes to assist in chemical reactions which destroy the oxidants or free radicals. Cypress essential oil is a moderate antioxidant, aiming to detox the body of free radicals that lead to disease.

Antibacterial

Cypress' antibacterial properties make it a powerful protectant against diseases produced by bacteria, such as oral, digestive and urinary tract bacterial infection. What's great is that, unlike some prescription drugs, Cypress has no ill effects on body wellness or on the healthy natural flora that exists within the stomach and intestines.

Antifungal

While bacteria and viruses are plenty evil, fungi commonly lead to the deadliest infections, whether external or internal. Your ears, throat and nose are the most likely to become infected by fungi, the infections of which can be both excruciating and unsightly. If left untreated, fungal infections can kill, as they may spread to the brain. Cypress essential oil protects against these infections and more and is particularly effective against skin infections.

Anti-inflammatory

External or internal inflammation can be reduced using Cypress essential oil. For instance, if you or your patient has swollen fingers from arthritis or a swollen knee from a sport's injury, topical application of Cypress essential oil may decrease irritation or redness, while also soothing the pain that accompanies inflammation.

Cytotoxic

Cypress essential oil has shown cytotoxic activity against cancer cell lines. This means Cypress is toxic to certain cancer cells, forcing these cells to lose membrane integrity and die rapid deaths through the controlled cell death program called apoptosis.

Sudorific

Cypress oil is sudorific, which means it induces perspiration. Periodic perspiration allows your body to release toxins, as well as excess water and salt. Sweating also clears the pores, because it opens the sweat glands. This supports the body's defenses against acne and other skin issues.

Sedative

As a sedative, Cypress sedates and calms by reducing anxiety, excitement or irritability. Though sedatives, alone, do not alleviate pain, they do calm the patient, making them less stressed and more compliant.

Antiseptic

The antiseptic activity of Cypress essential oil can be reaped topically, applied directly to wounds, or even through burning; the smoke from the oil may help destroy airborne germs. Topical use will help keep the wounds from becoming infections, support the body's natural function, and inhibit tetanus.

Astringent

For those who do not know what an astringent is, it's a chemical compound that shrinks body tissues, which means it can aid skin issues and irritations, everything from acne to insect bites. The astringent property of Cypress essential oil benefits everything from skin to hair to muscles to intestines. As an astringent, Cypress is an anti-agent, combating muscle loss through the ability to strengthen. This astringent property also means that diarrhea can be relieved through use of Cypress essential oil, as well as wound and cut bleeding.

Antispasmodic

The antispasmodic properties of Cypress oil make it beneficial to such surgical processes as colonoscopy, gastroscopy, and intraluminal-applied double-contrast barium enema.

Decongestant

As a decongestant, Cypress essential oil can alleviate nasal congestion in the upper respiratory tract.

Vasoconstrictor

Similarly, to the astringent property of Cypress, the oil's vasoconstrictor property supports the body's contraction of blood cells, which helps to cease excessive bleeding.

Diuretic

If you're looking to lose water weight and reduce blood pressure, Cypress essential oil is your agent. The oil stimulates urination, promoting not only the loss of water weight, but the loss of fats, uric acid, sodium, and other body toxins.

Hemostatic

A hemostatic promotes blood clotting, and so can be used to accelerate the clotting process when a person is bleeding profusely. Cypress essential oil does this by stimulating muscle, skin, gum, hair follicle and blood vessel contraction.

Hepatic

As a hepatic, Cypress essential oil supports the liver by managing bile discharge and promoting optimal liver function. The oil also helps to protect against liver infections.

Mucolytic

A mucolytic is a substance that helps dissolve large amounts of mucus, supporting proper breathing by clearing up the respiratory pathways. Cypress essential oil can thereby serve individuals who have coughs.

Common Therapeutic Uses

Traditionally used to enhance the body's defenses against respiratory issues, Cypress essential oil remains a significant support for overall wellness, protecting against several conditions that affect the respiratory tract. Cypress supports menstrual and post-menopausal wellness, while disinfecting and providing pain relief, amongst several other specialties. Let's take a closer look at the common uses for this oil.

Respiratory Issues

As a mucolytic and a decongestant, Cypress essential oil calms coughing by opening the airways. Bronchitis, congestion, asthma, sinusitis, cough, and other respiratory issues can be supported with Cypress essential oil, as the oil's anti-inflammatory and antispasmodic properties also promote a healthy respiratory tract.

Women's Wellness

Cypress can significantly benefit women at any age, due to its positive impact on menstruation and body image. Administering Cypress, particularly during periods of menstrual influx, can support the body's natural function by reducing heavy flow and relieving menstrual cramps. If you commonly experience painful or irregular periods, a Cypress application can be a helpful oil to have in your toolbox. Cypress essential oil also helps postmenopausal women by promoting self-image and reducing abdominal fat.

Liver Wellness

Cypress supports healthy liver function through its detoxification and hepatic properties. By clearing toxins through its sudorific activity, causing the body to sweat the bad out, function improves across all the body's systems. Cypress is also a hepatic, which means that the oil helps regulate bile discharge from the liver, promoting optimal liver function and protecting against liver infection.

Disinfectant

As a disinfectant, Cypress can be added to household cleaners to disinfect your home. The oil eliminates contamination, which means your household will be healthier overall, and will fall sick less often. Cypress can be used purely or blended with other oils to clean dishes, clothing, and practically any surface.

Candida Infections

The primary cause of urinary tract infection is Gram-negative E. coli, which is amongst the many bacteria and fungi studied against plant extracts. Cypress was discovered to be highly effective against E. coli, which means it can help inhibit UTI's, as well as support general urinary wellness.

Skin Care

Cypress oil is sudorific, which means it induces

perspiration. Periodic perspiration allows your body to release toxins, as well as excess water and salt. Sweating also clears the pores, because it opens the sweat glands. This supports the body's defenses against acne and other skin issues. The oil's astringent properties invigorate dull skin, while its detoxifying properties help cleanse and eliminate excess oil. Whether using Cypress essential oil to defy skin aging or to reduce adolescent skin issues, like pimples and acne, the antiseptic, sudorific, anti-inflammatory, and astringent properties are the best for skin issues, bar none.

Pain Relief

Cypress' anti-inflammatory qualities make it an effective pain reliever to be used in support the body's natural function against headache, sprains, injuries, wounds, scars, bruises, burns, and arthritis. It's a surefire aid to any sports muscle sprain or recovery pain from surgery.

Safety Precautions & Common Applications

Safety

Certain adverse effects may evolve when using pure essential oils. Some essential oils should not be used when pregnant, for example, as they may cause miscarriage. Allergic reactions, too, may occur, especially when applied topically. Always administer an allergy test before committing fully to topical application. When used with other medications, essential oils may react negatively. If you are on any current prescription medications or have a chronic illness, such as high blood pressure, epilepsy or liver disease, then researching the effects of essential oils against your own personal medical history will eliminate any potentially problematic issues.

Cypress has not been approved by the FDA for internal consumption and so should not be used as a dietary supplement. If you have sensitive skin, dilute heavily and test before extensive use. Otherwise, dilute 1:1 with a carrier oil. You can apply topically, diffuse, or use in other aromatic applications.

Blends

Oftentimes, essential oils are manufactured as blends of several pure oils. For instance, the Protective Blend of certain brands is a mix of cinnamon, clove, rosemary, and eucalyptus. This blend can be used to boost the immune system to help support colds, viruses and flus. The downside to blends is that the more oils added to the mix, the higher the probability your patient may react negatively to the blend if he/she is prone to allergies. There is also the possibility of phototoxicity when working with blends, particularly if they include citrus oils. Be sure to read your labels before administering.

Regardless of these possible effects, essential oils are a viable option for supporting several conditions. Those looking to support or maintain their own personal wellness, or that of their families', should become educated on the uses of essential oils, their natural remedies and the methods of application. Only then can you begin building your kit of essential oils for survival

Chapter 2:
Recipes for Cypress Essential Oil

In this chapter, we'll offer various recipes for Cypress essential oil, both for pure Cypress applications and blends. For pure applications, we've provided the appropriate dosage and method of administration to support specific ailments, from addiction to viral infections. When it comes to blends, herbalists and aromatherapists often combine Cypress essential oil with clary sage, bergamot, marjoram, rosemary, juniper, sandalwood, frankincense, pine, and lavender. We'll offer some fantastic blending options in the second half of this chapter.

Pure Applications

Aneurysm

To protect against aneurysm, dilute Cypress essential oil in a 1:1 ratio with a carrier oil and apply topically, massaging over the back of the neck, the forehead, and into the reflex points of the feet daily. For added support, diffuse throughout the room.

Arthritis

Support the body's natural defenses against the pain and inflammation of arthritis by diluting Cypress essential oil in a 1:1 ratio with a carrier oil and applying topically, massaging the oil into the joints.

Bacterial Infections

Combat bacterial infections by diluting Cypress essential oil in a 1:1 ratio with a carrier oil and applying topically over the affected area or massaging into the reflex points of the feet. You may also place a few drops in a bath or diffuse the oil for a similar effect.

Bone Spurs

Protect against bone spurs by diluting Cypress essential oil in a 1:1 ratio with a carrier oil and applying topically over the affected area two times daily.

Bunions

Rid your feet of bunion pain by diluting Cypress

essential oil in a 1:1 ratio with a carrier oil and applying topically over the affected area daily.

Bursitis

To help alleviate the pain and inflammation of bursitis, dilute Cypress essential oil in a 1:1 ratio with a carrier oil, then apply topically, massaging into the affected area.

Capillary Wall Strength

Strengthen your capillary walls by adding Cypress to your massage oil. You may also dilute Cypress essential oil in a 1:1 ratio with a carrier oil, then apply topically, massaging into the reflex points of the feet.

Carpal Tunnel Syndrome

Carpal tunnel syndrome can be eased by diluting Cypress essential oil in a 1:1 ratio with a carrier oil; then apply topically on the wrists, hands, and forearms, massaging into the affected area toward the shoulder, while placing a good amount of pressure on the muscles and tendons.

Catarrh

Relieve excess buildup in the nose and throat by applying one drop of Cypress essential oil directly over the nose and sinus areas. When using topically, avoid the mucus membranes and eyes.

Circulation Stimulant

Boost blood circulation by diluting Cypress essential oil in a 1:1 ratio with a carrier oil, then apply topically, massaging the application over the heart and into the arms and legs, towards the heart.

Concussion

Support concussion symptoms by diluting Cypress essential oil in a 1:1 ratio with a carrier oil; then apply topically, massaging the application into the soles of the feet and the back of the neck.

Connective Tissues

To support connective tissues, dilute Cypress essential oil in a 1:1 ratio with a carrier oil, then apply topically, massaging into the affected area and into the reflex points of the feet.

Control Issues

Whether you find yourself lacking self-control or attempting to dominate others, you may administer Cypress essential oil to stimulate or reign in control issues. Apply topically, after diluting it in a 1:1 ratio with a carrier oil. Massage the solution into the soles of the feet. You can also diffuse throughout the room to support this issue.

Diarrhea

If you're experiencing diarrhea, Cypress essential oil is a superb support. Apply topically by diluting the oil in a 1:1

ratio with a carrier oil and massaging it into the abdomen in a counterclockwise motion.

Dysmenorrhea

Dysmenorrhea, or painful periods, can be avoided by diluting Cypress essential oil in a 1:1 ratio with a carrier oil and applying topically over the lower abdomen, as well as into the ankles and the arches of the feet. You can also apply to a hot compress and press over the abdomen when experiencing painful cramps.

Edema

To relieve edema due to hot/humid weather, dilute Cypress essential oil in a 1:1 ratio with a carrier oil and apply topically for three days, once in the morning and once in the evening, to the outside of the leg, from the knee up to above the waist.

Endometriosis

To combat the pain of endometriosis, dilute Cypress essential oil in a 1:1 ratio with a carrier oil and massage into the lower back, abdomen, and into the reflex points of the feet three times daily.

Fear

To help eliminate unwarranted fear, dilute Cypress essential oil in a 1:1 ratio with a carrier oil and apply topically, massaging over the solar plexus and the heart. You can also administer aromatically, diffusing throughout the home or inhaling directly from the bottle.

Flexibility (Physical or Mental)

Enhance either physical or mental flexibility through administering Cypress essential oil. For physical enhancement, dilute Cypress essential oil in a 1:1 ratio with a carrier oil and apply topically, massaging over the affected area. For mental enhancement, diffuse throughout the room.

Flu

Support the body's natural defenses against the flu per its symptoms by diluting Cypress essential oil in a 1:1 ratio with a carrier oil; then apply topically, massaging it into sore muscles and joints, over the stomach, and into the soles of the feet multiple times, daily. You can also diffuse throughout the home to support general wellness during cold/flu season.

Oily Hair

Eliminate oily or greasy hair by placing a drop of Cypress essential oil in each single portion of shampoo and using as normal.

Grief

To uplift the spirit in a time of grief, diffuse Cypress essential oil throughout the home. You can also place a drop of the oil into your hands, rub your palms together, cup them over your nose, and breathe deeply in and out for several minutes.

Grounding

To help keep you grounded, place one drop of Cypress essential oil into your palm and rub your hands together. Place your hand over your nose and mouth and inhale. You can also apply topically, diluting the oil in a 1:1 ratio with a carrier oil and massaging into the reflex points of the feet.

Hemorrhoids

To relieve hemorrhoids, dilute Cypress essential oil in a 1:1 ratio with a carrier oil (or more for sensitive skin) and apply topically to the affected area.

Hiatal Hernia

Hernias can be targeted with Cypress essential oil by diluting in a 1:1 ratio with a carrier oil; then apply topically, massaging gently over the affected area.

Incontinence

To relieve incontinence, dilute Cypress essential oil in a 1:1 ratio with a carrier oil and apply topically, massaging into the abdomen once a day.

Lou Gehrig's Disease

Support the symptoms of Lou Gehrig's Disease by diluting Cypress essential oil in a 1:1 ratio with a carrier oil; then apply topically, massaging into affected area, the spine, the back of the neck and the reflex points of the feet three times weekly.

Lymphatic System Cleanse

To cleanse the lymphatic system, Cypress essential oil can be applied topically. Dilute in a 1:1 ratio with a carrier oil and massage your arms and legs toward the heart. Combine this application with healthy water intake.

Menopause

Support the body's natural defenses against menopausal symptoms by applying Cypress essential oil topically, diluting the oil in a 1:1 ratio with a carrier oil and massaging over the chest, lower abdomen, and into the soles of the feet. You can also diffuse throughout the home to maintain hormonal balance.

Menorrhagia

Support menorrhagia, or heavy/prolonged bleeding during menstruation, by diluting Cypress essential oil in a 1:1 ratio with a carrier oil and massaging over the lower abdomen and into the reflex points of the feet daily, during and between cycles.

Muscle Maintenance

To relieve muscle fatigue or help tone the muscles, dilute Cypress essential oil in a 1:1 ratio with a carrier oil and massage the solution into the affected area, toward the heart. You may also add a few drops to your massage oil or a hot bath.

Nose Bleeds

Alleviate nose bleeds by applying a single drop of Cypress essential oil over the nose and sinuses. You may also diffuse throughout the home if nose bleeds are chronic.

Pain

General chronic pain can be eased by diluting Cypress essential oil in a 1:1 ratio with a carrier oil; then apply topically, massaging over the respective reflex points of the feet in relation to the area of bodily pain or directly into the affected area.

Pleurisy

To combat the symptoms of pleurisy, dilute Cypress essential oil in a 1:1 ratio with a carrier oil and massage the solution into the chest once a day.

Preeclampsia

Protect against preeclampsia by diluting Cypress essential oil in a 1:1 ratio with a carrier oil and massaging into the reflex points of the feet. *Administer with caution during pregnancy. Ask your physician for support before use.

Prostatitis

To support the prostate, dilute Cypress essential oil in a 1:1 ratio with a carrier oil and apply topically, massaging over the affected area and into the reflex points of the feet on a regular basis.

Raynaud's Disease

Support the symptoms of Raynaud's Disease by diluting Cypress essential oil in a 1:1 ratio with a carrier oil and massaging it over the affected area and into the reflex points of the feet.

Retina Support

Strengthen and support the retina by applying a single drop of Cypress essential oil topically under the eyes and over the temples. Be careful to avoid getting oil in the eyes.

Rheumatoid Arthritis

To combat the pain and inflammation of arthritis, dilute Cypress essential oil in a 1:1 ratio with a carrier oil and apply twice daily, massaging the oil into the joints. You can also simply diffuse or steam two drops of the oil in a pan of water. Then remove the steaming pan from the stove, pour into a bowl, place a towel over your head and inhale. If you don't feel it's done its job the first time, you can reheat that same water and use it once more without adding more oil.

Skin Renewal

Renew and revitalize the skin by placing a drop of Cypress essential oil into your moisturizer or cleanser each time you follow your daily skin regimen.

Spasms

To relieve muscle spasms, dilute Cypress essential oil in a 1:1 ratio with a carrier oil and massage the solution into the affected area, toward the heart, and into the reflex points of the feet.

Stress

Combat stress by steaming two drops of Cypress essential oil in a pan of water, remove the steaming pan from the stove, pour into a bowl, place a towel over your head and inhale. If you don't feel it's done its job the first time, you can reheat that same water and use it once more without adding more oil. You can also diffuse throughout the room or place a drop onto your shirt collar for portable stress relief.

Stroke

Enhance the body's defenses against stroke by diffusing Cypress essential oil throughout the home or inhaling directly. You can also apply topically, diluting in a 1:1 ratio with a carrier oil and massaging into the temples, the reflex points of the feet, and the back of the neck.

Swollen Eyes

Relieve swollen eyes by applying a single drop of Cypress essential oil topically under the eyes and over the temples. Be careful to avoid getting oil in the eyes.

Toxemia

To relieve toxemia, you can apply topically, diluting Cypress essential oil in a 1:1 ratio with a carrier oil and massaging into the feet once a day or in a full-body massage once a week.

Tuberculosis

Tuberculosis can be targeted with Cypress essential oil, due to its ability to clear the airways, combat bacterial infections, and relieve inflammation. To apply topically, dilute Cypress in a 1:1 ratio with a carrier oil, then massage the oil over the chest and back and into the reflex points of the feet. You can also inhale directly or diffuse.

Urinary Infection

Support the body's natural defenses against urinary infection and promote healthy function by diluting Cypress essential oil in a 1:1 ratio with a carrier oil; then apply topically, massaging it over the bladder and kidneys. For added support, drink plenty of fluids.

Varicose Veins

Reduce the appearance of varicose veins by diluting Cypress essential oil in a 1:1 ratio with a carrier oil and applying topically to the affected area in an upwards stroke towards the heart.

Water Retention

To reduce water retention, dilute 1-3 drops of Cypress

essential oil in a 1:1 ratio with a carrier oil and apply topically, massaging over the affected area toward the heart.

BLENDS

Acne

Ingredients

10 drops Cypress Essential Oil

10 drops Lemon Essential Oil

5 drops Lavender Essential Oil

100 mL Carrier Oil

Directions

Target acne by combining all ingredients in a small glass jar or container and applying topically to the areas of concern.

Arthritic Pain Relief

Ingredients

1 drop Ginger Essential Oil

2 drops Cilantro Essential Oil

3 drops Cypress Essential Oil

2 Tbsps. Carrier Oil

Directions

Relieve arthritic pain by combining all ingredients in a small container. Tighten the lid and shake well. Apply topically, massaging into arthritic wrists or knees whenever you're in need of pain relief.

Cellulite Zapper

Ingredients

2 drops Cypress Essential Oil

2 drops Sage Essential Oil

4 drops Lemon Essential Oil

4 drops Cedarwood Essential Oil

5 drops Eucalyptus Essential Oil

2 ounces Carrier Oil

Directions

To reduce the appearance of cellulite, combine all ingredients in a small glass jar or container and apply topically to the areas of concern.

Circulation Stimulant

Ingredients

4 drops Cypress Essential Oil

2 drops Rosemary Essential Oil

2 drops Cilantro Essential Oil

2 drops Wild Orange Essential Oil

½ ounce Coconut Oil

Directions

To stimulate circulation, combine all ingredients in a small container, mixing until well blended. Apply topically to the ankles towards the heart.

Detoxification

Ingredients

2 drops Juniper Essential Oil

2 drops Lavender Essential Oil

2 drops Grapefruit Essential Oil

2 drops Basil Essential Oil

2 drops Cypress Essential Oil

30 mL Carrier Oil

Directions

To flush out toxins and boost circulation, combine all ingredients, blending well, and massage into the reflex points in the feet.

Emotional Soother

Ingredients

2 drops Cypress Essential Oil

2 drops Wild Orange Essential Oil

2 drops Frankincense Oil

2 drops Bergamot Essential Oil

Directions

To calm emotions and balance the psyche, combine all ingredients in your diffuser and diffuse as normal.

Female Fertility Rub

Ingredients

3 drops Ylang Ylang Essential oil

5 drops Eucalyptus Essential Oil

5 drops Lavender Essential Oil

5 drops Cypress Essential Oil

10 drops Basil Essential Oil

10 drops Frankincense Essential Oil

15 drops Geranium Essential Oil

15 drops Marjoram Essential Oil

25 drops Clary Sage Essential Oil

2 Ounces Carrier Oil

Directions

To improve chances of fertility, combine all ingredients in a small bowl, blending well. Massage into the reflex points of the feet two or more times a day. Store in a glass bottle.

Hemorrhoids

Ingredients

5 drops Geranium Essential Oil

1 drop Marjoram Essential Oil

1 drop Cypress Essential Oil

1 drop Lavender Essential Oil

1 Tbsp. Carrier Oil

Directions

To relieve hemorrhoids during pregnancy, combine all ingredients in a small bowl, blending well. Apply to the affected area then soak in a sitz bath for 10 minutes.

Hemorrhoids II

Ingredients

2 drops Clary Sage Essential Oil

2 drops Helichrysum Essential Oil

2 drops Geranium Essential Oil

2 drops Cypress Essential Oil

1 Tbsp. Carrier Oil

Directions

To relieve hemorrhoids during pregnancy, combine all ingredients in a small bowl, blending well. Apply to the affected area then soak in a sitz bath for 10 minutes.

Hepatitis

Ingredients

4 drops Basil Essential Oil

4 drops Myrrh Essential Oil

4 drops Cypress Essential Oil

8 drops Coconut Oil

Directions

To support the body's natural defenses against hepatitis, place all ingredients into a small bowl or container and blend thoroughly then administer topically, massaging into the liver and into the reflex points of the hands and feet.

Liver Tonic Support

Ingredients

2 drops Patchouli Essential Oil

2 drops Marjoram Essential Oil

2 drops Bergamot Essential Oil

3 drops Frankincense Essential Oil

3 drops Cilantro Essential Oil

4 drops Cypress Essential Oil

1 tsp Carrier Oil

Directions

To support healthy liver function, combine all ingredients in a small container and mix well. Every evening for up to two weeks, apply topically the area of the liver (right side of the body, below the ribs) and to the soles of the feet.

Lymphatic Salve

Ingredients

4 drops Cypress Essential Oil

3 drops Cilantro Essential Oil

3 drops Lime Essential Oil

3 drops White Fir Essential Oil

2 drops Patchouli Essential Oil

2 drops Rosemary Essential Oil

3 Tbsps. Coconut Oil

Directions

To relieve leg or feet swelling or edema due to hot/humid weather, combine all ingredients in a small bowl or glass container and mix well. Apply topically for three days, once in the morning and once in the evening, to the outside of the leg, from the knee up to above the waist.

Perineal Healing

Ingredients

2 drops Lavender Essential Oil

2 drops Cypress Essential Oil

Directions

Add ingredients to a sitz bath and soak for 10-15 minutes, three times daily.

Mental Clarity

Ingredients

6 drops Lemon Essential Oil

4 drops Rosemary Essential Oil

2 drops Cypress Essential Oil

1 tsp Carrier Oil

Directions

To clarify the mind, combine all ingredients and apply topically, massaging into temples and into the soles of your feet.

Muscular Pain Relief

Ingredients

6 drops Juniper Essential Oil

6 drops Lavender Essential Oil

4 drops Cypress Essential Oil

2 ounces Grapeseed Oil

Directions

To relieve muscle aches and pains, combine all ingredients in a small bowl or glass jar, blending well. Apply in a full-body massage or target the affected area.

Shaving Blend

Ingredients

2 drops Cypress Essential Oil

2 drops Lavender Essential Oil

2 drops Chamomile Essential Oil

2 drops Patchouli Essential Oil

1 Tbsp. Carrier Oil

Directions

For a close shave that naturally conditions the skin, combine all ingredients in a small bowl, blending well, and apply to the face before shaving as usual.

Smooth Skin Salve

Ingredients

6 drops Cypress Essential Oil

6 drops Geranium Essential Oil

¼ cup Coconut Oil

Directions

To make your skin smooth as silk, combine all ingredients in a small glass jar or container and apply topically to the areas of concern.

Chapter 3:
Cypress Essential Oil Studies

Many studies have been done on essential oils to uncover and prove their therapeutic qualities. In the case of the great number of Cypress studies, many of the properties attributed to the essential oil (noted in this book and elsewhere) are quite often validated through the research from accredited universities and published by reputable scientific journals. In this chapter, we'll discuss a small portion of these studies. It's important to note that research on essential oils is constantly evolving. Keep up with any recent research, as it may turn up even further valuable uses for these miracle oils.

Study 1 – Antimicrobial Properties

In this study published by *Complementary & Alternative Medicine*, the antimicrobial and antibiofilm effects of Cypress essential oil were examined, with the following results: "Cypressus sempervirens is a medicinal plant traditional, its dried leaves are used in treatment of stomach pain, diabetes, inflammation, toothache, laryngitis and as contraceptive...The present study was conducted to evaluate the in vitro antimicrobial, antibiofilm and determination chemical contents of the essential oil (Eo) and methanol extract from Mediterranean C. sempervirens L...The results presented here may suggest that the Eo and extracts of C. sempervirens possess antimicrobial and antibiofilm properties, and therefore, can be used as natural preservative ingredients in food and/or pharmaceuticals."

In this study, the Cypress essential oil and its constituents were evaluated, with results demonstrating that α-pinene, δ-3-carene, limonene, and α-terpinolene comprised most of the oil content. The methanol extract was shown to possess the highest antibacterial activity, with Klebsiella pneumonia, a Gram-negative bacterium that can be destructive to the human lungs, proven to be the most susceptible to the methanol.

These results indicate that the extracts from Cypress essential oil and the oil, itself, may be effective in pharmaceutical use and food preservatives as an active antibacterial agent.

Reference
http://www.ncbi.nlm.nih.gov/pubmed/24890383]

http://www.ncbi.nlm.nih.gov/pmc/articles/PMC4052795/

Study 2 – Antibacterial & Antifungal Properties

In this study published in *Ancient Science of Life*, the antibacterial and antifungal effects of Cypress essential oil were examined, with the following results: "The essential oil of leaves of various cupressus species Viz., C.glauca, C.funebris, C.lawsonia, C. macrocarpa & C. sempervirens have been studied for their antimicrobial activity against certain gram positive [B. subtilis, S.aureus], gram negative [E.coli, P.aeruginosa] and fungi (A.niger, A.flavus, C.albicans & A. fumigatus) using two fold serial dilution technique. Our results revealed that, all the species possess significant antibacterial & antifungal activities."

This study demonstrated the antifungal and antibacterial activity of Cypress essential oil on B. subtilis, S. aureus, E. coli, P. aeruginosa, A. niger, A. flavus, C. albicans and A. fumigatus. Let's go over each of these bacteria and fungi in turn.

Bacillus subtilis is a Gram-positive bacterium found in both soil and the human gastrointestinal. It is a safe bacterium, often used as a probiotic in those who are healthy. It may only cause disease in immunocompromised patients and very rarely causes food poisoning.

Staphylococcus aureus is Gram-positive bacterium. Although Staphylococcus aureus is part of the normal human skin flora and respiratory tract and is not typically pathogenic, those with compromised immune systems can potentially develop an infection from the bacteria. When it becomes pathogenic, S. aureus produces respiratory issues like sinusitis, skin infections, and even food poisoning.

Escherichia coli is another Gram-positive bacterium, which can cause serious food poisoning.

Pseudomonas aeruginosa is common bacteria found in water, soil, skin flora, and in man-made environments. The bacterium thrives on moist surfaces, and so can threaten the hospital environment by finding its home on medical equipment, like catheters, which may result in cross-infection. It is, for instance, the bacterium which causes hot-tub rash. P. aeruginosa also attacks immunocompromised patients, infecting the urinary tract, airway, wounds, burns, and resulting in blood infections.

Aspergillus niger is a fungus that causes black mold disease on some fruits and vegetables, like onions, apricots, grapes, and peanuts. A. niger is a common food contaminant, thrives in soil, and grows in indoor environments as well, which can cause wellness problems for inhabitants.

Aspergillus flavus is a pathogenic fungus appearing in

cereal grains, tree nuts, and legumes, during stages of harvest, transit, or storage. Many Aspergillus flavus strains produce compounds, called mycotoxins, which are toxic when consumed. A. flavus can also produce opportunistic human pathogens, causing aspergillosis, which may result in tuberculosis or ear, eye, nose, or nail infection in immunocompromised individuals.

Candida albicans develops as yeast and filamentous cells and can potentially cause genital and oral infections.

Aspergillus fumigatus is a fungus that causes disease in immunocompromised individuals. A. fumigatus creates colonies that become airborne and can compromise those with leukemia or AIDS, as well as organ transplant recipients, as it can become pathogenic and overthrow the weakly defended immune systems of these individuals.

The study's results demonstrated that all the Cypress species (cupressus sempervirens, included) showed significant antibacterial and antifungal activities against all the fungi and bacteria tested.

Reference
http://www.ncbi.nlm.nih.gov/pubmed/22435409]

http://www.ncbi.nlm.nih.gov/pmc/articles/PMC3330931/

Study 3 – Post-Menopausal Wellness

In this study published by *BMC Complementary & Alternative Medicine*, the effects of Cypress essential oil on the abdominal fat and body image of postmenopausal women were examined, with the following results: "The purpose of this study was to verify the effect of aromatherapy massage on abdominal fat and body image in post-menopausal women…The results suggest that Aromatherapy massage could be utilized as an effective intervention to reduce abdominal subcutaneous fat, waist circumference, and to improve body image in post-menopausal women."

The study involved two groups of women, a control and an experimental group. Each received a body massage treatment for one hour, once a week for six weeks. The women in the control group were massaged with grapeseed oil, while those in the experimental group received a Cypress-grapeseed blend. The study's objective was to evaluate the effect of aromatherapy massage on abdominal fat and body image in the subjects.

Data was collected pre- and post-test from both groups, including physical measurements and psychological wellness tests, and the results demonstrated that the waist circumference and abdominal subcutaneous fat were reduced more in the experimental group than in the control group. Body image had also improved more in the experimental group than in the control group. These results indicate that Cypress essential oil can be used in aromatherapy massage to improve body image and decrease waist circumference and abdominal subcutaneous fat in postmenopausal women.

Reference:
http://www.ncbi.nlm.nih.gov/pubmed/17615482]

Study 4 – Antioxidant, Anti-inflammatory & Anti-proliferative Properties

In this study, available on PubMed, the antioxidant, anti-inflammatory and anti-proliferative activities of Cypress essential oil were examined, with the following results: "Essential oils (EO) possess antimicrobial, anti-inflammatory, insect repellent, anti-cancer, and antioxidant properties, among others. In the present work, the antioxidant, anti-inflammatory and anti-proliferative activities of Moroccan commercial EOs (Citrus aurantium, C. limon, Cupressus sempervirens, Eucalyptus globulus, Foeniculum vulgare and Thymus vulgaris) were evaluated and compared with their main constituents...The antioxidant and anti-inflammatory activities of the EOs were plant species dependent and not always attributable to the EOs main components. Nevertheless, the EOs anti-proliferative activities were more related to their main components, as with T. vulgaris, C. limon, E. globulus and C. sempervirens."

This study examined Citrus aurantium, Citrus limon, Cupressus sempervirens, Eucalyptus globulus, Foeniculum vulgare and Thymus vulgaris essential oils. The objective was to compare the essential oils' antioxidant, anti-inflammatory and anti-proliferative activities with that of their main components. The study found that all oils demonstrated antioxidant, anti-inflammatory and anti-proliferative activities, but that the antioxidant and anti-inflammatory activities of the oils were not always directly attributed to the oils' main components, while the anti-proliferative activities were, especially in the case of Cypress essential oil. This likely indicates that the antioxidant and anti-inflammatory activities of Cypress are the result of the synergistic effect of all the oil's components, while its main components are responsible for the oil's anti-proliferative activities.

Reference
http://www.ncbi.nlm.nih.gov/pubmed/24868891]

Study 5 – Cytotoxicity

In this study published by *Cell Proliferation*, the effects of Cypress essential oil on human cancer cell lines were examined, with the following results: "The purpose of this study was to evaluate cytotoxic activity of Platycladus orientalis, Prangos asperula and Cupressus sempervirens ssp. pyramidalis essential oils and to identify active components involved in inhibition of population growth of human cancer cell lines...Our findings provide novel insights into the field of cytotoxic properties of essential oils. This study provided evidence on how cytotoxic activity of the oils is not always related to their major constituents…This opens a new field of investigation to discover mechanisms responsible for the observed activity."

The study evaluated the cytotoxic activity of several essential oils, including Cypress, on human cancer cell lines. The objective was to uncover the active cytotoxic components in the oils. The oil's antiproliferative activity was tested on amelanotic melanoma C32 cells, which is a type of skin cancer cell, and on renal cell adenocarcinoma cells, which is a cancerous tumor that occurs in the kidney.

Of all the oils tested, Cypress showed the highest cytotoxicity against the skin cancer cells. The chemical components found to be the most active against both cancer cell lines were terpenes, linalool, beta-caryophyllene and alpha-cedrol. Of these components, Cypress contains terpenes and linalool, which likely influence the oil's antiproliferative activity. However, like the previous study, the findings indicate that the cytotoxic activity of the oils is not always related to their major constituents and, thus, the synergistic effect of the entirety of the oil's components likely comes into play.

Reference:

http://www.ncbi.nlm.nih.gov/pubmed/19040575]

http://onlinelibrary.wiley.com/doi/10.1111/j.1365-2184.2008.00561.x/abstract]

Study 6 – Antioxidant Properties

In this study published by *Natural Product Research*, the antioxidant activities of Cypress essential oil were examined, with the following results: "In this study, supercritical fluid extraction (SFE) with CO2 and hydro distillation (HD) were compared as methods to isolate the essential oil from Cupressus sempervirens... Phenolic composition and antioxidant activity were also determined."

The study compared two extraction methods – supercritical fluid extraction with CO2 and hydro distillation – while also determining the oil's antioxidant activity. Cypress was shown to have antioxidant properties, and the supercritical fluid extraction method revealed more advantages than hydro distillation, including the extraction time and the yield, which was 34% better with SFE.

Reference
http://www.ncbi.nlm.nih.gov/pubmed/23316864]

http://www.tandfonline.com/doi/abs/10.1080/14786419.2012.755680?tab=permissions#.VPSLTeF9VCo]

Chapter 4:
The Ins & Outs of Essential Oils

Where do essential oils come from?

Plants and plant species naturally produce essential oils for various reasons, one being to draw pollinator insects to them, another being to repel invading organisms (bacteria, animals). A number of chemical compounds compose each plant's essential oil, and the combination of these compounds are specific to each oil, which then instills in the oil its own unique properties. Essential oils can be harnessed from all sorts of plant components, including flowers, leaves, bark, fruit, roots, and resin. For instance, cinnamon oil is harnessed from bark, lemon oil from the peel, and lavender oil from flowers. Certain plants can produce a few chemical variants of the same essential oil, which are acquired from different parts of the plant. Some of these parts produce a large amount of oil, while others produce just a smidgen. The oil's quality and potency depends upon a number of factors, including the subspecies of the plant, its soil conditions, the time of year and even the time of day it is harvested.

How are essential oils extracted?

Essential oils can be extracted from plants through various methods, including pressing, distillation, solvent and maceration. Let's take a brief look at each:

Pressing Method

Commonly used with citrus fruit, the pressing method extracts the oil through a technique which involves pushing the fruit peels through a press. Oily fruits and plants are best suited for this technique. Orange oil, for example, is extracted from orange skins through the pressing method.

Distillation Method

This technique harkens back to the days of moonshiners, as the same sort of method used to create strong liquor can be used to extract essential oils. Using a still, boiled water and plant materials will create steam which is then cooled by coils and condensed into a combination of water and oil. This combination does not mix, so the oil can then be extracted from it.

Solvent Method

Through a multi-step process, certain plant and flower oils can be extracted using alcohol and other solvents, which extort the essential oil from the plant materials.

Maceration Method

When a "carrier," fixed oil, or lard is mixed with the plant material and set out in the sun, over a period of time, the carrier oil is infused with the plant's essence. Heat sources, other than the sun, are often used to speed the process. Throughout the process, more plant material is added to produce a more potent oil.

How do you use essential oils?

Although some studies about the effectiveness of essential oils are conducted by small companies or even individuals, a number of them are conducted by the food and cosmetic industries. In general, the pharmaceutical industry shows next to no interest in herbal medicine, primarily because there are few options to patent such products. As such, the product's lack of profitability results in a lack of research funding. Regardless, the historical uses of essential oils tell us what we need to know: these oils have been effectively administered for centuries. The therapeutic qualifications of essential oils can be plotted in the survival of the human race across cultures and generations.

Another reason that studies on essential oils have not resulted in much conclusive evidence as to their overall effectiveness is because definitive results are sometimes difficult to prove, as the quality of each batch of oil can vary for a number of reasons. One is that essential oils are impossible to standardize. As mentioned above, even the slightest variance in soil conditions and the time of harvesting – as well as innumerable other factors – will produce a different product quality and potency. In addition, essential oils are often obtained from various species of the same plant; Eucalyptus radiata and Eucalyptus globulus can both be used in the making of therapeutic-grade eucalyptus oil and as a result, they may have slightly different properties and degrees of strength or effectiveness.

Just as there are a number of methods by which to extract essential oils, there are a number of methods to administer them therapeutically. The variety of chemical compounds in each essential oil means that their benefits and applications also vary across the board. Below are a few of these methods.

Topical Administration

Direct application of many essential oils works like a sponge, as skin absorbs chemicals and other things (like sunlight, for instance). Topical application is best when you want to clear up an ailment on the skin's surface, or in the underlying muscle tissue. When applying topically, either massage the oil into the skin, or simply dab on the skin for therapeutic results. Combine the essential oil with a carrier oil for topical use in order to dilute its potency. This is safer, as the oil is very concentrated. Support the body's defenses against rash or muscle pain in this manner, but you should always test a patient for allergies before applying. Adverse effects are produced by natural chemicals as much as synthetic ones; poison ivy, for example.

To test for allergens, place a drop or two on your patient's inner forearm. If a rash develops within 12 to 24 hours, then the patient is allergic. In addition, phototoxicity – sun exposure resulting in an exacerbated burn – may be an issue when citrus oils are applied topically. One must proceed with caution when applying essential oils using this method.

Inhalation Therapy

Commonly known as "aromatherapy," this essential oil application is effective for inner ailments, like sore throat or cold. In a steaming bowl of distilled or sterilized water, add a few drops of essential oil and with a towel over the head, bend over the bowl and inhale. The towel captures the vapors, making the technique even more effective. Essential oils can also be placed in a diffuser, or potpourri, throughout a room to produce somewhat diluted therapeutic effects.

Ingestion

When using this method proceed with caution. Direct ingestion of essential oils must be monitored and applied in small doses that are diluted in a tablespoon or more of any carrier oil – olive oil, for example. If unsure of dosage amounts, make a tea with the relevant herb instead. Although the effects of this diluted use may be weaker, this application is a better alternative than an overdose of essential oils.

What are the general benefits of using essential oils?

Supplement for Prescription Drugs

One practical benefit for using essential oils is of course, their supplemental nature; which is the ultimate reason to educate yourself on their administration and to begin stockpiling an essential oil supply. One of the potential threats of economic, or social collapse, is the lack of resources, and primarily the inability to procure prescription drugs. As such, finding suitable alternatives should be a priority when preparing for the worst.

Their portability is also a major bonus when it comes to survival prepping. The fact that these ultra-concentrated oils take up little-to-no space makes toting them to a shelter all the simpler should the need arise. Because essential oils are highly concentrated, the application used in most methods of administration requires only a drop or two of oil, which means that a tiny bottle will be long-lasting.

Cost Effective Supplement

Though money may be the last thing on your mind when it comes to prepping for a survival situation (money may even be obsolete in the event of social collapse), it is worth noting that the expense of essential oils pales in comparison to prescription drugs. In fact, whether or not you are forced to survive on essential oils due to a lack of prescription reserves, in some cases, you might consider supplementing prescriptions with these inexpensive alternatives regardless. Essential oils are a cost effective supplement to prescription medicine.

No Expiration Date

Another benefit of essential oils is that they do not expire, nor do they have "proper storage" requirements. A number of medicines and medicinal products must be replaced every couple of years; this sets essential oils ahead of the pack when it comes to shelf life.

Versatility

Essential oils also offer great versatility. Apart from providing wellness benefits, essential oils can be repurposed for household and hygienic applications. For instance, if looking for something that might serve dental hygiene needs in a time of crisis, thieves oil is the go-to essential oil. In order to maintain the skin's tone and condition, frankincense and lavender will do the trick; the latter also serves as sunscreen, so it can protect against sun damage as well.

When it comes to the house or shelter, use essential oils to deodorize, which will come in handy in a disaster scenario where things might start to smell bad due to lack of proper utilities and care. For example, after the 2011 tsunami and the subsequent nuclear reactor meltdown in Japan, a nurse named Risa Nakahira used essential oils to deodorize and sanitize putrid public bathrooms in overpopulated evacuation facilities. As relief workers searched for survivors, often wading through debris and decay, Nakahira also deodorized their boots and masks using essential oils. The possibilities of these natural oils are endless.

They are also versatile when it comes to the range of patients they are capable of supporting. The wellness of everyone from great grandfather to infant baby can be fortified with the aid of essential oils in the appropriate dosage. They even come in handy when supporting the wellness of livestock or pets. From teething infants to dementia in the elderly, from teenagers with acne to dogs with urinary tract infections, essential oils can serve any patient with nearly any ailment.

Conclusion

Now that you know all about what essential oils can do for you, you can start to assemble a kit of essential oils to support your anti-aging goals. Visit www.oilsclass.com to claim your free bonus video training.

The various benefits of essential oils and their properties are countless. To build your own kit, first focus on acquiring the essential oils which may bear more relevance to your aging issues or the potential health threats within your environment that may be contributing to premature aging. shot, and you'll quickly be inspired to produce your own creative products with essential oils on your own terms.

DISCLAIMER AND/OR LEGAL NOTICES: Every effort has been made to accurately represent this book and it's potential. Results vary with every individual, and your results may or may not be different from those depicted. No promises, guarantees or warranties, whether stated or implied, have been made that you will produce any specific result from this book. Your efforts are individual and unique, and may vary from those shown. Your success depends on your efforts, background and motivation.

The material in this publication is provided for educational and informational purposes only and is not intended as medical advice. The information contained in this book should not be used to diagnose or treat any illness, metabolic disorder, disease or health problem. Always consult your physician or healthcare provider before beginning any nutrition or exercise program. Use of the programs, advice, and information contained in this book is at the sole choice and risk of the reader.

www.ingramcontent.com/pod-product-compliance
Lightning Source LLC
Chambersburg PA
CBHW062102280526
45788CB00003B/1322